UNDERSTANDING

COLLAGEN

AND BENEFITS

A Comprehensive Guide to Understanding its Major Targets, Key Points, and Focus on Enhancing Your Health and Beauty

DR. LACEY MICHELLE

Disclaimer:

The information provided in this book is for general informational purposes only and is not intended as medical advice.

Readers are encouraged to consult with a qualified healthcare professional for any health concerns or questions.

The author of this book is not affiliated with any individual, website, organization, or products mentioned within.

This book does not endorse or promote any specific brands, services, or external entities. Any references made are purely for illustrative purposes and should not be construed as endorsements.

Readers are responsible for their own decisions and should conduct their own research before making any health-related choices.

Any liability resulting from the use of this information, whether direct or indirect, is disclaimed by the author and publisher.

Contents

Supplementing with Collagen

We explore the amazing world of collagen in the pages that follow. Collagen is a necessary protein that keeps many facets of our health and well-being in check. This book is your entire guide to understanding collagen, especially when it comes to supplements. It covers the vast range of applications of collagen in supporting the health of your skin, joints, and digestive system as well as its potential for anti-aging, weight management, and recovery after exercise. In let's start by delving into the basics of collagen.

Definition of Collagen. We'll explore the fundamentals of collagen, its enormous significance, and the various varieties in this first chapter, which will prepare you for the in-depth discussion of collagen supplementation that comes next.

Sources of Collagen Learn where collagen comes from naturally and why collagen supplements are getting more and more well-liked. We'll look at the several ways you can get this essential protein.

Advantages of Collagen Supplements This chapter explores the several advantages of collagen supplements, such as better skin, support for joints, and increased health of the muscles, nails, intestines, and hair.

Types of Collagen Supplements Learn about the distinct characteristics of the several types of collagen supplements that are available, including beverages, powder, capsules, and collagen peptides.

How to Pick the Best Collagen Supplement There are several things to take into account while choosing the best collagen supplement. This chapter offers helpful advice on how to make an informed decision about anything from dosage and time to reading labels.

Collagen Supplements and Anti-Aging Discover how collagen helps maintain age-related bone health, improve skin suppleness, and lessen wrinkles in our search for youthful vitality.

Collagen and Exercise Recovery Examine how taking collagen supplements can help with joint support, muscle recovery, and tendon and ligament health, which makes them a vital tool for athletes.

Collagen Supplements and Weight Management Learn how collagen supplements can help with metabolic augmentation, hunger control, and the maintenance of a nutritious diet.

Collagen and Digestive Health This chapter explores the relationship between collagen and digestive health, including issues such as irritable bowel syndrome, leaky gut syndrome, and the possibility of gut repair.

Collagen and Medical Issues This section examines the impact of collagen on several medical issues, such as osteoporosis, joint disorders, arthritic ailments, and wound healing.

Collagen and Beauty Goods: From topical uses to its integration into cosmetics, we explore the significance of collagen in beauty goods.

Combining Collagen with Other Supplements To Get the most out of your health regimen, discover how collagen works in concert with other supplements including vitamins, minerals, and various proteins.

The Science Behind Collagen Supplements Learn how collagen functions and examine the most recent studies and clinical trials that attest to its effectiveness.

Side Effects and Precautions Learn about possible drug interactions, allergies, and safety measures to take when taking collagen supplements.

Including Collagen in Your Daily Routine

Offers helpful advice on how to incorporate collagen into your daily routine, along with meal plans, smoothie and drink recipes, and more.

The Future of Collagen Supplements:

In this last chapter, we take a look ahead and examine new developments and trends in collagen products, providing a fascinating preview of what's to come in the collagen supplement industry.

This book is a great tool for anyone looking to improve their health, discover the benefits of using collagen supplements, and keep up with the most recent developments in the industry. Our investigation into collagen may be useful to you whether you want to enhance joint health, improve the quality of your skin, or just lead a healthier life. Now let's go off on this fascinating adventure to discover the mysteries of collagen supplements.

CHAPTER ONE

Knowing About Collagen

Describe Collagen. One essential protein that the human body uses as a structural building block is collagen. It is the most prevalent protein in animals, including humans, and is essential to the upkeep of the suppleness, strength, and integrity of different tissues and organs.

This fibrous protein supports the skin, bones, tendons, ligaments, and more; it can be compared to the glue that holds the body together.

Although collagen is present in every part of the body, the amount varies depending on the tissue and its intended use.

The Significance of Collagen in the Body Collagen is significantly more important to the body than just a structural element. It benefits a person's general health and well-being in several ways. Most importantly, collagen is necessary to keep skin healthy. By keeping the skin firm and supple, it helps to avoid sagging and wrinkles. Furthermore, by maintaining cartilage integrity and fostering joint flexibility, collagen is essential for maintaining joint health. Collagen is essential for the health of bones, hair, nails, and several internal organs in addition to its function in maintaining skin and joints.

Furthermore, because collagen is an essential part of the gut lining, it also has an impact on the digestive system. It contributes to overall gut health by keeping toxic chemicals from the digestive tract from leaking into the bloodstream. Since collagen plays a key role in the production of scar tissue, its significance in the body is demonstrated by its role in wound healing. In conclusion, collagen is a complex protein that plays a major role in maintaining the body's structural integrity, general health, and functionality.

Types Of Collagen Collagen

is a protein that comes in different forms, each having unique properties and roles inside the body. It is not a single, homogenous protein. Although collagen comes in at least 28 varieties, Type I, Type II, and Type III are the most widely used varieties.

Type I Collagen: Found in the skin, bones, tendons, and ligaments, this type is the most prevalent. It is in charge of preserving these tissues' structural integrity and giving them tensile strength. Because of its importance to skin health, it is frequently the subject of numerous collagen supplements and cosmetics.

Type II Collagen: Mainly found in cartilage, type II collagen is essential to joint health. It is crucial for preserving joint flexibility and averting diseases like osteoarthritis since it contributes to the construction and cushioning of joints.

form III Collagen: Commonly present in blood arteries and different organs such as the liver, lungs, and spleen, this form of collagen is frequently found in conjunction with Type I collagen. For these tissues and organs to be elastic, type III collagen is essential.

Different bodily sections also contain less frequent forms of collagen, such as Type IV and Type V, each of which has a distinct purpose. When thinking about collagen supplementation, it's critical to understand the different types of collagen because some types may be advantageous for treating particular health issues.

CHAPTER TWO

Sources Of Collagen:

Synthetic and animal sources are both possible for collagen. The most popular source of collagen in food and dietary supplements is collagen obtained from animals.

Collagen can be extracted from animal bones, skin, and connective tissues and used to make collagen supplements. Fish is another good source of collagen, especially the skin and scales, which are high in Type I collagen.

Collagen supplements are also suitable for people with dietary restrictions or ethical concerns about animal products because they can be made from synthetic or plant-based sources. Rather than giving the body direct collagen, these plant-based collagen substitutes frequently include components like hyaluronic acid, vitamins, and minerals to encourage the body's natural manufacture of collagen.

Collagen is an important protein that serves a variety of vital purposes in the body. Selecting the best collagen supplement or including foods high in collagen in one's diet requires knowledge of the benefits of collagen and the various available forms.

Furthermore, collagen comes from both plant- and animal-based sources, providing options for those with different dietary needs and preferences.

Health And Collagen

A structural protein called collagen is essential to many facets of human health. It is the most prevalent protein in the human body and may be found in the skin, bones, tendons, and cartilage, among other tissues. The possible health benefits of collagen supplements have made them more popular in recent years.

We shall examine the numerous functions of collagen in preserving and enhancing various facets of health in this article.

Function Of Collagen In Skin Health

The beneficial effects of collagen supplements on skin health are among their most well-known advantages. The structural element of the skin that gives it flexibility and moisture is collagen.

Collagen production naturally declines with age, causing fine lines, wrinkles, and drooping skin to appear.

By increasing the amount of collagen in the skin, collagen supplements may help minimize the look of aging and give the skin a more youthful appearance. Collagen is an important ally in preserving skin that is vibrant and healthy since it may also aid in wound healing and scar reduction.

Collagen For Healthy Joints

The connective tissues in our joints, such as the ligaments and cartilage, are made primarily of collagen.

Joint tissues may deteriorate over time as a result of severe wear and tear or the aging process itself. Joint pain and osteoarthritis are two disorders that may result from this. It is thought that collagen supplements help maintain joint health by supplying the building blocks required for cartilage regeneration and repair. Consuming collagen regularly may help reduce joint pain and increase mobility, making it a desirable choice for people looking to preserve or improve their joint health.

Collagen And The Recovering Muscle

Collagen supplements are frequently used by athletes and fitness enthusiasts to help with muscle rehabilitation and performance. A major component of muscle and tendon tissues is collagen.

Eating collagen may aid in improving muscle strength, lessen discomfort in the muscles, and speed up the healing process after exercise. Furthermore, some studies indicate that collagen supplements may increase the body's synthesis of creatine, a substance that powers muscle contractions, enhancing both muscle repair and function.

Collagen And Systemic Absorption

Although its function in digestive health is less well understood, collagen plays a critical role in preserving the integrity of the gut lining. To stop toxic compounds from entering the bloodstream, the gastrointestinal tract needs a robust and unbroken barrier.

Collagen helps heal damaged intestinal walls and gives the lining of the stomach its structural integrity. After taking collagen supplements, some people with ailments including leaky gut syndrome and irritable bowel syndrome have experienced improvements in their symptoms. This shows that by supporting gut integrity, collagen may have a beneficial effect on digestive health.

Growth Of Collagen And Bones

Collagen is also essential in the bones, another important area. Collagen strands give bones strength and resilience by acting as a framework for minerals such as calcium. Bone density can decrease with age, raising the risk of osteoporosis and fractures. Supplementing with collagen may aid in maintaining bone strength and density.

According to studies, collagen can promote the growth of bone-forming cells, preserving bone health and possibly lowering the incidence of fractures in older people.

Collagen And The Health Of Hair And Nails

Collagen is good for the body's outward features, such as hair and nails, in addition to its inside components. The main protein found in hair and nails is called keratin, and the synthesis of keratin depends on collagen. Supplementing with collagen may result in stronger nails and thicker hair.

 Moreover, it can aid in preventing hair breakage and brittle nails. A lot of people use collagen in their cosmetic regimens to get healthier, more vivid nails and hair.

Collagen supplements are becoming more well-known for their ability to improve a range of health issues.

Collagen may provide a natural and efficient answer for any of your goals, including improving the appearance of your skin, reducing joint discomfort, enhancing muscle recovery, promoting digestive health, maintaining strong bones, and enhancing the quality of your hair and nails. Before incorporating collagen supplements into your daily routine, you should, however, speak with a healthcare provider to be sure they are suitable for your unique set of medical requirements.

CHAPTER THREE

Supplemental Collagen

A protein called collagen is essential for preserving the structural integrity of the skin, bones, tendons, and cartilage, among other tissues in the human body.

Collagen production in the skin gradually decreases with age, resulting in problems including wrinkles, joint pain, and decreased skin suppleness.

Collagen supplements are a popular remedy for these symptoms. There are many different kinds of collagen supplements, and they are thought to help with joint function, skin health, and other things.

But it's critical to comprehend the many kinds of collagen supplements, how to use and dose them, as well as any possible hazards or adverse effects from consuming them.

Various Supplement Forms For Collagen

There are many different types of collagen supplements on the market, but the most popular ones are collagen peptides, collagen protein, and collagen capsules.

Collagen is hydrolyzed to create smaller, easier-to-absorb molecules, which are called collagen peptides. They can be added to foods and beverages and are frequently found in drink mixes and powders.

Conversely, collagen protein is rich in amino acids and comes from animal sources, such as bone broth.

An easy approach to consuming collagen orally is with collagen capsules. The form that is chosen depends on personal tastes and the particular advantages that the person is looking for.

Dosage And Use Of Collagen

Depending on a person's demands and goals, there are differences in the right amount and application of collagen.

The recommended range of doses is usually 2.5 to 15 grams per day, but the exact amount should be determined by speaking with a healthcare provider.

To improve absorption, collagen supplements are frequently taken on an empty stomach. Some people like to take them in the morning or right before bed.

It may take many weeks to months to observe changes in skin, hair, or joint health, so consistency in use is crucial.

CHAPTER FOUR

Selecting An Appropriate Collagen Supplement

Choosing the best collagen supplement is an important choice. It's important to take into account the source of collagen, whether it is from fish, poultry, porcine, or cow. Supplemental collagen is frequently labeled with a type, such as type I, type II, or type III, based on the source of the collagen and the intended uses.

For instance, type I collagen is frequently utilized to maintain the health of the skin, but type II collagen is linked to joint support. It's also important to look for additives, fillers, and allergies on the ingredient list. To guarantee quality and safety, it is recommended to select products from reliable producers who have undergone independent testing.

Possible Adverse Reactions And Hazards

Although collagen supplements are thought to be safe overall, there may be some adverse effects.

There have been isolated reports of gastrointestinal distress, including bloating and diarrhea, especially at high dosages. People who are allergic to the collagen's source—for example, shellfish allergies in the case of marine collagen—should proceed with caution.

Furthermore, it is imperative that you speak with a healthcare professional before beginning a collagen supplement program if you have any medical concerns, are pregnant, or are breastfeeding a baby.

Always take prescription medications as directed, and stop using medication if side effects arise.

Products For Beauty With Collagen

Collagen is a common component in many different types of cosmetic products and is not just found in oral supplements.

Collagen is frequently used in creams, serums, and masks to enhance the elasticity, moisture, and general appearance of the skin. It's crucial to remember that there is disagreement over the efficacy of collagen given topically.

Due to their size, collagen molecules may find it difficult to pass through the skin's protective layer and reach deeper layers where they are required.

However, collagen-infused cosmetic products are a subset of the larger skincare and anti-aging product market that accommodates personal preferences, and they may offer benefits only noticeable on the surface.

Collagen In Certain Diet Plans

In recent years, collagen supplements have become increasingly popular as more individuals use them in their diets for a variety of health and aesthetic advantages. The most prevalent protein in the human body, collagen, is essential for preserving the structural integrity of our connective tissues, skin, and joints.

Although the body naturally produces collagen, as we age, our ability to generate it tends to decline, which can result in wrinkles, joint discomfort, and other indicators of aging. People frequently use collagen supplements to treat these problems, and there is curiosity about how they fit into particular diets like the Paleo, Keto, vegan, and vegetarian diets.

The Paleo Diet's Use Of Collagen

Often called the "caveman diet," the Paleo diet is based on foods that our predecessors would have eaten in the Paleolithic period. It avoids grains, legumes, and processed foods in favor of whole foods, lean meats, fish, fruits, and vegetables. Since collagen is an animal-based protein, it naturally fits in with the Paleo diet's tenets. Collagen-rich foods such as skin, tendons, and bone broth are recommended in this diet.

People who follow the Paleo diet also frequently utilize collagen supplements to increase their intake of collagen. These dietary supplements come from animal sources, including the collagen found in chicken, beef, or fish. They complement the Paleo diet's emphasis on fostering general well-being and treating particular health issues like joint pain and skin aging by supporting joint health and enhancing skin suppleness.

On The Keto Diet, Collagen

The keto diet is a high-fat, low-carb eating regimen that induces ketosis, a state in which the body uses fat rather than carbs as its main energy source.

The Keto diet places restrictions on foods high in carbs, which are frequently a major source of collagen in the diet. This restriction begs the question of how people following a Keto diet can consume enough collagen.

Collagen supplements are a useful complement to the Keto diet to treat this issue. They provide a practical means of boosting collagen consumption without sacrificing the macronutrient balance of the diet. Collagen peptides provide the necessary amino acids needed for the body to produce collagen and can be added to a variety of Keto-friendly dishes and drinks.

Collagen in Diets of Vegetarians and Vegans

Vegetarian and vegan diets are plant-based eating regimens that forgo foods originating from animals. The fact that animal tissues contain the majority of collagen poses a problem for people who adhere to these diets. Although plant-based diets are very beneficial to health, they may be low in collagen, which can cause issues with joints and aging skin.

Nonetheless, there are collagen supplements on the market that are suitable for vegans. The plant-based ingredients used to make these supplements, such as seaweed and a variety of fruits and vegetables, can supply the amino acids required for the synthesis of collagen.

While they might not give collagen directly, they aid in the body's production of it, which helps vegans and vegetarians address particular issues related to their health and appearance.

Depending on personal dietary preferences and health objectives, collagen supplements can be included in specific diets including the Paleo, Keto, Vegan, and Vegetarian diets.

Comprehending the various sources and types of collagen supplements is essential for making well-informed decisions and guaranteeing compliance with the tenets and limitations of the selected diet.

Collagen supplements can be a useful adjunct to these particular diets, addressing specific health and beauty concerns while supporting dietary preferences, whether for improved joint health, skin elasticity, or overall well-being.

CHAPTER FIVE

Collagen And Recipes

The potential benefits of collagen supplements for healthy skin, hair, nails, and joints have made them more and more popular in recent years. These supplements can be simply added to a variety of dishes to increase their nutritional content.

They usually come in powder, pill, or liquid form. Recipes that increase collagen have become popular among those who want to get healthier all around. We'll talk about the ideas behind collagen-boosting dishes in this session, such as smoothies and snacks made with collagen.

Recipes For Boosting Collagen

Recipes for collagen-boosting ingredients are made using delicious items that also help the body produce and maintain collagen. The structural protein collagen is essential for connective tissues, joints, and skin suppleness. The natural production of collagen in our bodies declines with age, thus replenishing it becomes increasingly important.

These recipes frequently include components high in the building blocks of collagen, and amino acids such as glycine, proline, and hydroxyproline.

To promote collagen synthesis, foods like bone broth, poultry, fish, and certain plants like kale and spinach are frequently used in these recipes. Individual preferences can be catered to when creating collagen-boosting dishes, whether they are for a hearty meal, a nutritious snack, or a morning smoothie.

Collagen-Based Drinks

Smoothies with collagen are a well-liked option for people looking for a nice and easy method to add collagen to their daily regimen. Collagen powder is a common addition to these smoothies because it has no taste and no odor, making it simple to mix with other ingredients. Collagen powder can be mixed with veggies like spinach or kale and fruits like bananas, mangoes, or berries to make a nutrient-dense, collagen-boosting drink.

Collagen smoothies frequently contain additional components like yogurt, almond milk, or even coconut oil in addition to fruits and vegetables. These components not only improve the flavor but also add extra nutrients that support the development of collagen and healthy skin. Smoothies containing collagen are an adaptable choice for individuals leading hectic lives, as they may be quickly and healthily ingested for breakfast.

Snacks With Collagen

Snacks enriched with collagen can both satiate your palate and give the advantages of collagen supplementation. These can be anything from homemade energy bars to candy with collagen.

For instance, collagen-infused gummies are an easy and enjoyable way to reap the health advantages of collagen while indulging in a tasty pleasure.

Collagen powder can be added to recipes for protein bars, homemade granola, or even desserts to make collagen-infused snacks. These delectable and nutritious snacks are a great choice for anyone trying to improve the health of their skin, hair, and joints because they frequently include collagen along with other components like nuts, seeds, and honey. These snacks are a good source of collagen in addition to being a healthful substitute for typical, frequently less nutrient-dense snacks.

Collagen supplements can now be included in diets through dishes that promote collagen, such as smoothies and snacks made with collagen. In addition to being delicious, these dishes may help with joint support, stronger hair, and better skin health. People can discover collagen-boosting recipes that suit their dietary needs and preferences by experimenting with different ingredients and flavors, which will ultimately improve their general well-being.

CHAPTER SIX

Typical Myths Regarding Collagen

As a nutritional supplement, collagen, a protein that is found in large amounts in our skin, hair, nails, and connective tissues, has become more and more well-known in recent years.

However, there are a few widespread misunderstandings and fallacies about collagen that call for more research.

A common misconception is that taking collagen supplements can instantly make your skin seem better.

Collagen is necessary for healthy skin, but the body can only use so much of it when it is ingested.

Instead of directly replenishing lost collagen, the majority of research shows that collagen supplements work better to support the health of the skin by encouraging the body to produce new collagen. It's critical to set reasonable expectations for the instantaneous aesthetic benefits of collagen supplementation.

Another myth is that taking collagen supplements will aid in burning fat or losing weight. Some people think collagen can function as a fat burner or increase metabolism.

Nevertheless, this assertion is unsupported by any scientific data. The main function of collagen is as a structural protein; it does not affect metabolism. Collagen supplements by themselves are not a significant factor in the complex process of weight management.

Another prevalent misunderstanding regarding collagen is the idea that all collagen supplements are made equally. In actuality, there are various kinds of collagen supplements—Type I, Type II, and Type III, for example—and each has a distinct function in the body. Skin, hair, and nails are the main tissues that contain Type I collagen, whereas cartilage has Type II collagen. Skin and blood arteries contain type III collagen. Selecting the kind of collagen supplement that best suits your health objectives is crucial if you want to get the most benefits from it.

The idea that collagen supplements are suitable for vegans or vegetarians is another misconception that has to be busted.

The majority of collagen comes from animal sources, especially marine and bovine products. It presents a problem for people on plant-based diets.

Nonetheless, several businesses are attempting to create plant-based collagen substitutes that have similar properties.

While these substitutes don't contain collagen, they are made to encourage the body's natural creation of collagen without utilizing materials produced by animals.

Furthermore, there's a myth that collagen supplements can heal or treat several illnesses, including osteoporosis and arthritis.

Although collagen is essential for the health of bones and joints, it has little effect on the treatment of these disorders.

In certain situations, collagen supplements may help maintain joint health and lessen joint discomfort, but they shouldn't be used in place of conventional treatments that doctors have recommended.

Research And Studies In Science

Because of its popularity, scientists are studying collagen more thoroughly to determine its possible advantages and disadvantages.

Supplementing with collagen has been demonstrated in studies to improve skin health. Collagen peptides, for example, have been shown in studies to improve the suppleness, moisture, and general look of skin. These outcomes are linked to increased skin health as a result of stimulating the skin's production of collagen.

Research into collagen's function in joint health is another topic of interest.

According to certain studies, collagen supplements may help people with diseases like osteoarthritis feel less pain in their joints and have better joint function.

Since collagen is a necessary component of cartilage, taking supplements may help maintain the integrity of the cartilage and lessen joint inflammation.

Research on the possible advantages of collagen for gut health and muscle rehabilitation is also ongoing, in addition to its effects on skin and joint health.

Collagen may lessen the signs of digestive issues and support a healthy gut lining. Collagen supplementation is well-liked by athletes and fitness enthusiasts since it may also help with muscle regeneration and recuperation.

Even while collagen supplements are becoming more and more popular and may have several health benefits, it's crucial to distinguish fact from fiction when thinking about using them. While collagen can help with gut, joint, and skin health, it is not a miracle weight-loss aid or a panacea for a host of ailments.

Our comprehension of collagen's impacts will probably deepen with further research, offering more precise recommendations on how to employ it to preserve and enhance general health.

CHAPTER SEVEN

References And Achievements

Testimonials and success stories are seen as effective marketing strategies and are used extensively in the promotion of collagen supplements. People who have taken collagen supplements often talk about their own experiences, showing how these products have improved their lives.

These testimonies, which provide actual examples of the advantages of collagen supplements, are crucial in fostering trust among prospective customers.

Numerous testimonies regarding collagen supplements demonstrate the various ways in which these products have improved people's lives.

Due to collagen's function in boosting skin hydration and maintaining the structure of the skin, many people have noticed improvements in their skin's elasticity and reduction in wrinkles.

These first-hand reports frequently highlight how collagen supplements can help with the outward indications of aging.

Moreover, anecdotal evidence frequently reveals the beneficial effects of collagen on joint health.

Because collagen is an essential component of cartilage, testimonials often describe how taking supplements of collagen has reduced joint pain, improved mobility, and enabled people to lead active lives.

These tales are especially pertinent to people who have osteoarthritis or other similar illnesses.

Beyond appearance and physical well-being, collagen supplements are linked to improvements in nails and hair.

After adding collagen to their regular regimens, users have reported experiencing stronger nails and thicker, glossier hair.

This is because keratin, the protein that makes up hair and nails, is influenced by collagen.

To put it briefly, endorsements and case studies play a crucial role in bolstering the efficacy of collagen supplements. These first-hand accounts motivate anyone thinking about using collagen supplements by illuminating how collagen can improve individual lives.

First-Hand Accounts Of Collagen Use

The range of people who utilize collagen supplements is reflected in their varied experiences with them.

A large amount of our skin, bones, and connective tissues are composed of the protein collagen, which has been linked to numerous health advantages. Adding collagen to everyday activities has been associated with observable benefits in overall well-being, according to numerous reports.

Collagen supplements are a common way for people to improve the appearance of their skin since they promote moisture and improve suppleness. A more youthful complexion and fewer wrinkles may arise from this. Collagen supplements have also been reported by those with skin disorders like eczema or acne to have helped them have clearer, healthier skin.

The effect of collagen on joint health is another recurring element in firsthand accounts. Because collagen is an essential component of cartilage, people who have joint pain or stiffness frequently find relief from their symptoms by taking collagen supplements. The significance of collagen in sustaining an active and pain-free lifestyle is emphasized by these tales.

Another important component of individual collagen experiences is the state of one's hair and nails. Numerous people have mentioned having stronger, more glossy nails and hair, and some have even noted faster-growing hair. These enhancements are largely due to collagen's effect on keratin, the protein that makes up hair and nails.

Some people have reported that collagen has a favorable effect on their general vitality and energy levels in addition to its physical effects. Although collagen's primary function in the body is structural, some users say it gives them more energy, possibly as a result of better metabolism and nutrition absorption.

These first-hand accounts demonstrate the many advantages of supplementing with collagen and provide strong arguments for people to think about adding collagen to their daily routines.

The Impact Of Collagen On Lives

Numerous testimonials demonstrate the potential for collagen to have a profoundly positive impact on people's lives.

These modifications go beyond simple physical adjustments and can include boosts to self-esteem, general health, and standard of living.

Increasing self-esteem is one of the most prevalent ways collagen transforms people's lives. The improved condition of the skin, hair, and nails that collagen supplements frequently produce might boost one's self-esteem.

People say they feel better about the way they look, which improves their confidence and social relations.

For people who experience joint discomfort or arthritis, collagen's importance in maintaining joint health can change their lives. Many times, users discover that they can move again and do things they previously believed were impossible. Their quality of life and mental health are also improved, in addition to their physical health.

Collagen can be a game-changer for people who have been dealing with brittle nails or hair loss. Reviving one's hair and nails can help people feel more confident and normal about their appearance, which could have a profound impact on their lives.

Personal accounts have also mentioned collagen's beneficial effects on gut health, as it may help thicken the gut lining. Better digestion, fewer dietary allergies, and an all-around healthier and more comfortable life can result from this.

Collagen has a positive effect on general health, including heightened vitality, improved sleep, and more energy. Increased energy and better mental clarity have been noted by users, which has significantly impacted their daily routines and productivity.

Collagen has the power to transform lives by improving physical health, elevating self-esteem, and fostering general vigor and wellness. These profound adjustments highlight the importance of collagen supplements in the lives of numerous individuals.

Conclusion

The effectiveness of collagen supplements has been demonstrated by numerous testimonies and success stories, which have contributed to their enormous rise in popularity. Experiences with collagen personally demonstrate the variety of ways that it can improve people's lives. Collagen has transformed many lives by promoting joint mobility, healthy skin, and better-looking hair and nails.

Stories of how collagen has improved people's lives go beyond its obvious health benefits. They also include heightened self-worth, assurance, and general well-being. Collagen's importance in people's lives is further compounded by its impact on energy levels, digestion, and mental clarity.

Together, these firsthand accounts and individual experiences highlight the many advantages of collagen supplements. Collagen supplementation has the potential to positively impact health, even if individual outcomes may differ. In the world of dietary supplements, collagen's ability to support improved health and quality of life is becoming more widely acknowledged as more people share their experiences.